How To Lose Weight Without Working Out

HTeBooks

Disclaimer

This book is designed to provide condensed information. It is not intended to reprint all the information that is otherwise available, but instead to complement, amplify and supplement other texts. You are urged to read all the available material, learn as much as possible and tailor the information to your individual needs.

Every effort has been made to make this book as complete and as accurate as possible. However, there may be mistakes, both typographical and in content. Therefore, this text should be used only as a general guide and not as the ultimate source of information. The purpose of this book is to educate.

The author or the publisher shall have neither liability nor responsibility to any person or entity with respect to any loss or damage caused, or alleged to have been caused, directly or indirectly, by the information contained in this book.

Table of Contents

How Will This Book Help You?

A lot of people want to lose weight but rarely have the time for routine exercises or a well-planned healthy diet. However, it's NOT TRUE that you have to control your life with military precision in order to lose weight. The fact is that weight gain happens due to the accumulation of small, seemingly inconsequential habits that we have in our daily lives.

This book is meant to help you unlearn those bad habits while learning the small, inconsequential yet *helpful* ones that can result to weight loss. By the end of this book, you will become aware of your small weight-gain habits, discard them, and replace them with small, effortless weight-loss habits.

The best part about this book is that you'd be able to shed the pounds without going through extensive and rigorous workouts or incredibly difficult diets. In fact, you won't even feel a thing – except your skinny jeans as it becomes looser and looser on your hips!

Read on and find out exactly how this book can make this happen!

You're Not Hungry

"Appetite has really become an artificla and abnormal thing, having taken the place of true hunger, which alone is natural. The one is a sign of bondage but the other, of freedom"

- Paul Brunton, The Notebooks of Paul Brunton

In the old days, people ate when they needed to – the scarcity of food didn't leave much for indulgence. Nowadays however, food is everywhere and unfortunately, it is the most commonly used stress-reliever for most people. Feeling sad? Eat! Feeling bored? Eat! Most people aren't even aware of the extent of their eating habits, believing that they're eating properly but not really counting those extra bits of chocolate they snuck in when no one's looking.

That's why the first step for weight loss without working out is simple: control your diet, starting with the sheer amount of the things you eat.

Signs You're Not Really Hungry

The problem with the body is that it can fool you into thinking you're hungry when in truth; you actually need to fill a specific need. This is why before you open the fridge thinking to satisfy your hunger, it's best to take a step back and ask yourself first: am I really hungry? Here are some signs that your stomach is really fake-growling.

Specific Food Request

A first and common sign of fake-hunger is the specificity of your food request. Real hunger doesn't identify between different food types – as long as it's edible, you will eat it – if you're really hungry. If you happen to be imagining a perfectly glazed doughnut however while ignoring the fruits and vegetables in the fridge, chances are your stomach is just faking it.

Stomach Not Growling

A growling stomach is probably the strongest indicator of hunger. Once you hear sounds emanating from it, you'll know that it's been a long time since you last ate. Of course, it's not usually a good idea to wait until your stomach is making some noise before eating, but paying close attention to what your stomach *feels* like (empty, full, heavy, bloated) should give you a good idea on the status of your hunger pangs.

Instantaneous Hunger

Hunger is not instantaneous. You can't be full one moment and hungry the next, rather, the need for food should creep up on your as the body slowly uses up the food you've previously eaten.

Clock Says Otherwise

If you just ate 15 minutes ago, there's no way you can be hungry again. Typically, the human body experiences hunger in the morning, noon, and night time, hence: breakfast, lunch, and dinner. Some small hunger pangs may be felt around 9AM and 3PM – upon which you'd probably take a snack break. If you're seeking food at any time other than those mentioned, your body is just fooling you into thinking its hungry.

Still with Energy

Hunger usually leads to physical and emotional weakness. You'll find yourself becoming irritable and having a hard time moving around. Of course, it's important to note that this may not always be a sign of hunger. People who are on a high fat and sugar diet often feel sluggish or "heavy" due to the imbalance of their dietary consumption. It's best if you can distinguish between lethargy from a bad diet versus hunger weakness. If not, a low energy might bear less weight as a sign of hunger.

If even just two of these signs are present, it's best to walk away from the fridge right now! This is not actual hunger but rather, your mind fooling you into thinking you need more food. Now the question is, what do you do to distract yourself from giving in to the temptation? The next Chapter should help.

*Create a daily eating schedule. Eat only during those specific times of day.

How to Kill Fake Hunger

"Remember, you are not a heavy person trying to slim down. You are a trim, health person learning how to reemerge."

-Celso Cukierkorn

After discussing the existence "Fake Hunger", the next question would be – how do you kill this problem? Even if you *know* that you're not really hungry, the pangs are still there – which means that eventually, you'll find yourself giving in. Don't! There are ways to successfully stamp down the feeling and "fool" your body into thinking you've eaten. Here are some tips on how to do this:

Drink a Glass of Water

In some cases, "thirsty" and "hungry" become intertwined in the brain, making people think that they need food when all they really need is a tall glass of water. Therefore, when you start feeling those hunger pangs – go straight to the kitchen and pour some water down your throat. Wait at least 5 minutes...are you still hungry? Guzzle another glass and wait for 5 more minutes. If you're still feeling the same hunger then this is your "go" signal to actually eat something. More often than not however, the hunger pangs stop right there. The beauty of this technique is that for really hungry people, drinking a glass of water can actually make their stomach grumble, a sure sign of hunger. For those who aren't hungry, this helps fill the stomach and ensures that if they *do* eat, they'll consume fewer amounts of food.

Wait 15 Minutes

In most cases, 15 minutes is all it takes for your body to "forget" the hunger. This is because fake hunger is often instantaneous yet temporary. One minute, you have this very powerful urge to eat a donut and after 15 minutes or so, you won't even remember wanting a donut so badly.

Distract Yourself against Boredom

This works well with the 15-minute wait, allowing you to pass the time without watching the clock. Distraction can be in many forms, depending on what would hold your interest the longest. In most cases, simply refocusing the brain's attention is enough to stop your stomach from feeling fake hunger. Studies show that in most cases where people overeat, they are usually driven to it because they have nothing else to do, hence the frequent trips to the fridge to see what's available. It helps if you keep your day occupied with tasks or chores, therefore leaving no room for boredom.

Fighting Stress

It is often said that food is the most abused anxiety drug – which is why people who are often under a lot of stress find themselves eating every few minutes. For most, the taste and feel of food is a source of comfort, regardless of whether they feel full or not. This is often coupled with inactivity since a depressed spirit rarely wants to move. Obviously, the end result is rapid weight gain. So what do you do if stress is your main problem?

Exercise is the most underutilized anti-depressant, but that doesn't mean you have to instantly go out for a jog. Remember, we're trying to lose weight without workouts –so a different alternative to stress might become necessary. Following are some of the 'anti stress' techniques you can try out that don't involve eating or excessive physical activity:

Drink Tea

Chamomile tea is one of the most effective ways for you to relax. If this isn't to your liking, almost any other type of tea would do particularly lemon and green tea. Prepare them whenever you feel yourself becoming stressed.

Massage and Acupuncture

Individually, massage and acupuncture can offer stress relief as it targets specific areas of the body that are "locked" or experiencing tension. At least one of these every week should ensure that you end your working days relaxed with no massive appetite to deal with.

Sleep

Sometimes, the best way to handle nagging cravings and stress at the same time would be to sleep. Most people who use this technique find that when they wake up, their cravings tend to disappear. Not only that, but did you know that sleeping actually burns off more calories than watching TV?

Of course, those are just few of the techniques you can use to fight stress. It really depends on what works for you so make sure to check out different methods until you find the one you want.

*Bring a container of water with you wherever you go and take a sip whenever you experience cravings.

Easy Dietary Changes for Weight Loss

"Food is an important part of a balanced diet"

- Fran Lebowitz

Knowing how to kill fake hunger often won't cut it if you're looking to shed pounds quickly in a healthy way. It's important that you also take the time to create and follow a balanced diet to ensure that your body is getting all the nutrients it needs to stay strong. Unless you eat fast food for breakfast, lunch, and dinner however – a complete revamp of your daily diet might not be necessary. More often than not, simple dietary changes are the only things you'll have to do in order to lose weight. The great thing about these small 'steps' is that they're so simple, making them practically effortless to follow. That being said, following are the small techniques you can try out.

Warm Water in the Morning

Drink a glass of warm water in the morning before taking anything else. Two glasses of water would be best, but you can start with just one glass until you're used to the sensation. Doing so on an empty stomach helps with the digestion and ads up to your daily quota of 8 glasses. You'll find that after drinking, your stomach will grumble and you might find a need to go to the toilet – which is actually a good thing. Wait 30 to 60 minutes before eating or drinking your coffee. Some individuals also like to add a few slices of lemon into the mix, or perhaps a few teaspoons of freshly squeezed lemon juice. This has been proven to help speed up metabolism.

Water Before Eating

If you're going to settle down for a meal, it's a good idea to drink a glass of water first. This not only helps the digestion but partially fills your stomach so that you won't eat as much. Taking sips every few bites also helps tremendously in keeping your appetite in check.

Make Your Veggies Easy

The main reason why people eat so much junk food (aside from the fact that they taste great, of course) is the fact that they're so easy to eat. All you have to do is open a pack and start munching – so why not use the same technique for your fruits and vegetables. Apples and grapes are easy, but if you're partial to pineapples then make sure to purchase small, bite-size ones that you can put in a convenient to-go container. Baby carrots, carrot sticks, and sliced cucumbers are also perfect as snacks, providing you that 'crunchy' feeling that satisfies the stomach. Try preparing all these at night at a leisurely pace before sealing them all in an air-tight container inside the refrigerator. This way, you can just pop in a few in your mouth whenever you feel the need to chew on something.

Go Brown

White is not the natural color of most food items such as sugar. In most cases, these white food have gone through extensive processing in order to be commercial-ready, causing them to lose their natural color. Unfortunately, along with the color they also lose vital nutrients while taking in all sorts of chemicals used for the process. This is why if you want to lose weight, it's best to shift to natural and colorful food items such as green, red, orange, and brown. Their natural colors indicate that very little processing has been done, which means that most of their nutrients are still intact.

Eat Slow and Hot

This is a common problem nowadays when people only have less than 30 minutes to eat their breakfast and lunch. What happens is that they shove in spoonfuls of food in their mouth without really keeping track of how much they're eating. The problem here is that you eat food so quickly, the stomach doesn't have sufficient time to "register" that it is full. As a result, your body might have had enough to eat but your brain hasn't gotten the message yet – causing you to feel like you're still hungry. The solution – eat more slowly. By savoring your food one morsel at a time, the stomach finds it easier to register the food and signals the brain correctly when it's finally full. Studies also show that eating your food while it's hot can boost the "fullness" effect on the body – not to mention it forces you to eat slowly.

Love the Protein

Protein is a wonderful way to boost muscle growth – but it's also known to help a person feel fuller, faster. According to studies, swapping your carbohydrate diet with protein also helps with weight loss, specifically using eggs instead of say – a bagel or a donut. In the study, those who swapped their unhealthy breakfast for eggs experienced 65% more weight loss than those who didn't.

NO Diet Food

Some industries today are at their peak because they market to the dieting population. Often sold as "diet food", these prepackaged products claim to be low-fat, low-calorie, and low-everything which makes them "perfect" for people who want to lose weight. Don't believe the hype – anything that comes prepackaged and can last for more than a week is instantly suspect and should not be considered "healthy". Come to think of it, avoid all types of diet supplements as well. Remember: you want to lose weight in a healthy manner.

Juice Up!

If you're not fond of munching on carrot sticks, you might like drinking carrot juice better – or perhaps a combination of several vegetable and fruits. It really doesn't matter what your juice combination happens to be: as long as it doesn't come in a can or bottle, you're good to go! The great thing about juicing is that you can keep it in the fridge for some time and it won't go bad on you, but not too long though! For example, if you really don't have the time to fix breakfast, try juicing up your favorite combination at night and just drink it up in the morning!

No Soft Drinks

Some food items can be eaten in moderation – but some of them should be avoided at all costs. Soft drinks fall under the latter category and can provide absolutely no help to your body, aside from the good taste. Carbonated drinks are full of sugar and are the number one reason why people gain weight. If you drink at least one 500ml bottle of carbonated drink a week – that's already too much. Ditch this and opt for less-sugary fares. Water is always best but if you really need something with flavor, fruit drinks would work (but not necessarily healthier). Always follow up a sugary drink with water.

Wine in Moderation

It's generally accepted that alcohol is chock full of calories and should therefore be avoided if you want to start shedding the pounds. However, this only works if you drink several glasses a day. One glass after a meal however would be perfect, boosting your metabolism plus giving you that extra 'kick' that would let you go to sleep peacefully. Opt for red wine – it might have more calories, but the metabolic boost it provides is more than worth it. Keep in mind though, this only works in moderation.

Go Salsa

The most common comment made by dieters when switching to fruits and veggies is the bland taste of the food. For the most part, that's true because you've gotten used to the flavor-enriched servings of processed food items. However, you'll find that in time, the food starts to become tasty and you'll actually appreciate the natural flavor and texture of the food. In the meantime though – go crazy on the condiments! Not mustard or mayonnaise but rather, salsa! The calorie savings when using this particular condiment is significantly better than ketchup and mayonnaise plus the taste is something you can definitely get used to! Spoon it on everything and make sure you always have a ready supply.

Slimming Coffee

Skip the Starbucks coffee or any caffeine drink with loads of sugar. Go for black coffee or something with just a small teaspoon of sugar. You'll find that this not only helps jerk you awake better, but the calorie count is also lower.

*Always have carrot sticks ready in the fridge and bring some with you at work to munch on.

Working Out Without the Work

"When people tell me they can't afford to join a gym, I tell them to go outside; the planet Earth is a gym and we're already members. Run, climb, sweat, and enjoy all the natural wonders that is available to you."

- Steve Marboli, author of Unapolegitcally You: Reflections on Life and Human Experiences

When the word "exercise" is spoken, this usually brings forth images of men and women in tights, doing a run with earphones stuck in their ears. Or perhaps, you see people milling about in the gym, running on the treadmill and lifting weight – but is this exercise really looks like?

Exercise is defined as: an activity that requires physical effort.

This means that *any* form of physical activity can be considered an exercise – even if it's just you getting out of bed in the morning. The trick however is to maximize these 'exercises' so that they become equivalent to a gym visit while still molding perfectly with your lifestyle. So how exactly do you work out without working out? Here are some activities you can integrate in your daily routine that wouldn't feel like you're 'exercising'.

Taking the Stairs

Start by skipping the elevators and taking the stairs instead. This can get you where you want to go while providing you with excellent buns. A slow and steady climb will help but if you really want to get the heart rate going, it's best to climb up rapidly and feel the burn of your thighs and calves. The great thing about this is that you don't have to go down at the very moment – you just need to get to the office for a much needed rest. If you think you've had enough, it's always possible to take the elevator to your floor after a few flights.

Walking to Work

Walking to work is also another wonderful example of getting where you want to go without spending some of your hard-earned cash. In fact, walking helps you save on gas or at least the cost of commute. Of course, this might not always be a possibility, for example, your home might be too far away. If it's viable however, then do it! No need to do it daily – three times a week (MWF) should do nicely.

Drying Clothes the Old Fashioned Way

Nowadays, we tend to use the handy-dandy dryer to dry the clothes – which is perfect if you need to wear something quickly. For weekly laundry however, it's usually best to hang your clothes out to dry – allowing you to stand up, walk around and stretch those muscles as you pin clothes to the clothesline. It doesn't seem like much, but hanging clothes and taking them down after they're dry can burn hundreds of calories. The best part is that sun-drying is completely free with your clothes smelling fresher than ever.

Walking after a Meal

Sitting down after a meal hinders digestion, even if you manage to drink a glass of water afterwards. The solution: stand up and do some light walking after eating so that your stomach doesn't get "pinched" and it can continue working as needed. A good way of utilizing this time efficiently is by washing the dishes after a meal – after everything's been tidied up, your stomach should feel OK enough to sit down.

Sauna it Up

Saunas are wonderful ways to relax while losing all that excess fluid that's floating around your body. A lot of people have managed to lose weight through regular sauna as the heat helps with the removal of toxins in the body. Possible the best thing about saunas is the fact that they lead to better, smoother, and healthier looking skin.

Play Your Jam

Admit it – you also do an impromptu performance when your favorite song starts playing. This might seem like fun and games, but combining your favorite playlist with several household chores can actually make you more energetic, promotes physical movement and essentially gives your body a good workout while uplifting your mood. Make sure you have a playlist of some of your most favored songs and have it ready at all times.

Do What You Love

Sports can be incredible on the body but since you're having fun while doing it, it doesn't really count as a form of exercise. If there's any kind of sport you love doing – like badminton and swimming, then make a point of doing those at least twice a month! Find a badminton body or sign yourself up for the local pool for some frolicking and swimming. You'll find that sports don't just work towards weight loss but also helps develop the muscles and give you that incredibly toned body.

Housework

Housework can be a wonderful way to start shedding the pounds, a few decimal points at a time. It doesn't matter what kind of cleaning you happen to be doing: all of them works wonders. Dusting, throwing out the trash, fluffing the pillows, vacuuming the carpet, and various other forms of housework can help you work a few ounces of sweat. This might not seem like much, but totaled together – you're probably looking at more than 100 calories burned!

Now, there are lots of things that fall within the "housework" category. If you think this actually burns very little, you might be surprised! Here's a chart of specific housework's and the approximate amount of calories they burn for the average individual.

Housework	15 Minutes of Work
Sweeping floors	39
Mopping	43
Washing dishes (standing)	22
Cooking	17
Vacuuming	43
Carrying groceries	111
Child care	34

*Create a list of activities/chores that you can easily do manually without the aid of machinery or appliances. Do them.

Strengthening Your Willpower

"Enjoy losing weight. Enjoy eating healthy, delicious food. Do not wait until you reach your destination to feel good. Take as much happines and joy as you can from your weight loss journey."

- Harry Papas

The fact is that no matter how "small" these steps happen to be, you'll come to a point when your willpower wavers. You'll find yourself craving something or eating huge amounts of a particular food. This is understandable – especially if you're just starting out. Here's a step by step approach on how to deal with your craving-hunger-eat situation:

Step 1: Determine if you're feeling real hunger or not.

Step 2: If you're feeling fake hunger, utilize the techniques used to kill it.

Step 3: If you're experiencing real hunger, use the techniques offered on the chapter "Easy Dietary Changes for Weight Loss"

Step 4: If you still feel hungry or still craving food, start doing some of the suggestions offered in the chapter "Working Out Without the Work"

Step 5: If nothing still works, giving in to the craving is inevitable. However, that doesn't mean you'll have to consume as much as your stomach will allow. In this chapter, we'll talk about ways on how to boost your willpower.

Keep a Visual Reminder

A visual reminder gives you something to check out whenever you feel your willpower wavering. It can be a picture of you in your thinner years, or perhaps the picture of a model that has the kind of body you want. The important thing is that you don't sink into despair whenever you see this reminder but rather, it should inspire you into pushing forward with your goals.

Why Are You Doing This?

If you have a specific reason for attempting weight loss, always remind yourself of this reason whenever you feel yourself wavering. Are you doing this to look good for a wedding party, a reunion with friends, or do you simply want to look good when wearing a fashionable dress? It really doesn't matter what your reason happens to be – as long as it can fuel your willpower, then it will definitely help.

Keep it Small

Have both minor and major goals. One of the top reasons why people deter from their diet is because they have such big goals that their determination flags halfway through. If you're thinking to lose 50 pounds, try by targeting at least 4 pounds of weight loss every week. This way, you can measure every week and find out if you're meeting your weekly weight loss goal. Every pound lost at the end of the week throws fuel into the fire, allowing you to become more focused on the goal.

Willpower is a Muscle

Willpower is a muscle and the more you exercise it, the more capable you become of resisting temptation. This is why if you find yourself craving a generous slice of chocolate cake, don't shrug your shoulders and think: it's just for today. Every time you give in, you lose a little bit of willpower until you find yourself no longer sticking to your restrictions. Utilize will power at all times and always stop yourself before plunging in.

Of course, in the previous chapter, we've talked about giving in to the cravings once in a while so you're probably thinking – isn't this advice contradictory? How can I give in to the cravings while exercising willpower at all times? The next paragraph should tell you how.

Give In On Schedule

Simply put, give yourself a time and place to give in to these cravings. Assign a specific day indulge on sweet, high-fat food items. Typically, people choose Saturday or Sunday for this day, but this isn't always a good idea. Instead, you should opt for a weekday for your cheat day (Monday to Friday). This way, you'd consume less unhealthy food items because you'll be too busy with work. Assigning a weekend for cheating usually means you'd eat the whole day, significantly doubling your consumption. This technique works well as a sort of portion control.

Failed? Repeat!

Don't worry – people don't expect you to do this perfectly in just one go. If you've failed, then accept the mistake and move on. The important thing here is that you *don't give up.* Having a strong support system composed of friends and family also works wonderfully well and makes it easier for you to stay true to a healthier lifestyle.

*Whenever you feel your willpower being tested, take a deep breath and count to 3. Slowly let it out, this time counting backwards from 3 to 1. Repeat.

Small Things that Affect Your Weight Loss

"Weight loss is a sum of all your habits – not individual ones"

- Helen M. Ryan, 21 Days to Change Your Body

Most people are of the assumption that weight loss only covers two factors: what you eat and what you burn off during physical activity. The fact is that although this is the main *formula* to attain calorie deficiency, there are actually small habits that can significantly affect your goal. People don't really see these as related to weight loss but with careful study, you'll find that they actually fuel the fire of overconsumption and laziness. Here are the small things you'll need to avoid or practice in order to experience weight loss:

Watch the Clock

Studies have shown that erratic eating habits usually lead to faster weight gain and slower weight loss. This is because the body is confused about the exact time you're providing it with energy, causing it to become erratic with storage and calorie burns. The simplest solution here would be eating on time. You might think that postponing lunch until 3PM is no big deal as long as you get the food, but this might be the quickest way to weight gain.

Sleeping Schedule

Tiredness is often mistaken for hunger – which is why it's important that you are NEVER tired during the day. Obviously, the best way to make this happen is by getting 8 hours of sleep every 24 hours. It's been noted that people who work at nights tend to gain more weight – which can be due to the sudden change in eating-sleeping pattern. If you are one of these people, then it's important to treat your night time as if it was day time. For example, if you go to work at 8PM then you should wake up around 6PM and eat your "breakfast". Lunch would be around 12midnight and so on and so forth. Just make sure that you sleep at least 8 hours daily.

Size and Color of Your Plates

Believe it or not, the size and color of your plates actually affect your appetite in a very subconscious manner. Studies show that red and yellow enhances the appetite while blue inhibits it. Hence, if you want to go on a "subconscious" diet, it's probably time to switch your plate sets into the color blue. As for the size, large plates prompt people into filling them up which obviously leads to larger portion sizes. If you keep those plates small however, you'll find yourself unconsciously eating smaller and smaller amounts of the same food.

Menstrual Cycle

A common problem with most women is that with menstrual cycles comes the unbelievable craving for specific food items coupled with this extreme reluctance to move around. Even if you're not on a diet or exercising regularly, menstrual cycles can throw a huge crimp in your well-controlled lifestyle. A good way of battling this problem for women is by drinking green tea or black tea. This helps ease away the pain of discomfort of menstruation, removing the bloat you feel in your stomach and most importantly – it helps balance your palate so that you don't find yourself craving too much sweets.

No More TV Dinners

It's practically a routine for most people nowadays to eat in front of the television. Though it's definitely enjoyable, what you don't realize is that watching TV while eating makes it virtually impossible for you to keep track of your portion sizes. More often than not, individuals overeat when they watch television. The solution: turn off the TV and enjoy your meal the way you're supposed to. Eat only in the dining room with the entire ensemble that comes with it. Now, this might seem like too much for a single-person dinner, but you'll find that the action is actually very meditative, allowing you to become ready for dinner. By enjoying every morsel and experiencing every bite, you'd be able to eat slowly and therefore receive your brain's "I am full" signal as soon as the stomach sends the message.

One Hour after Dinner

Going to bed right after dinner is bad. Once you go to sleep, your metabolism slows down which basically means that everything you ate will likely turn into fat. Prevent this from happening by waiting at least an hour before going to bed. Two hours would actually work best but if you're tired – then go for it! Use the allotted one hour to mentally prepare yourself for sleep, taking a long shower, getting into your most comfortable pajamas, drinking tea and so on.

Your Clothes

Yes – the things you currently wear are definitely affecting your weight loss efforts. If you have lots of loose clothes, start throwing them away or perhaps putting them in a safe place in the attic. Loose clothes usually causes people to lose track of their weight loss efforts – simply because they feel comfortable in what they're wearing and feel like it's OK to still grow into these clothes. Instead, start buying tighter and tighter clothes – small enough so that you'd feel them touching your belly. Unconsciously, slowly shrinking your clothing collection prompts you into losing weight so that you'd continue to fit into them. It's like a reverse weight loss technique!

*Eat on time and only in places where you're supposed to eat.

How to Apply What You've Learned?

Diet and exercise aren't the only things that predict your weight gain and weight loss. After reading this book thoroughly, you now know that practically everything you do has an impact on your current weight. That being said, it's crucial for you to condense everything you've found out through this book into useful, actionable goals that would take you one painless step at a time to the body you've always wanted. Here are just some suggestions on how to apply what you've learned in this discussion.

Maintain a schedule for your meals and snacks.

Move more often.

Time yourself before giving in to cravings.

Take a deep breath whenever you're tempted – a clear mind helps you reaffirm that will power and make it easier for you to say "NO"

Have a mantra that you can repeat over and over again as a reminder.

Sip water continuously throughout the day.

The fact is that there are so many strategies you can utilize after reading this book to the last Chapter. As long as you understand the concept, you'll be in the position to make the small yet helpful changes that would shed the pounds one by one. Good luck!

www.ingramcontent.com/pod-product-compliance
Lightning Source LLC
Chambersburg PA
CBHW061947280526
45787CB00004B/1751